KIDNEY-FRIENDLY DIABETIC RECIPES

Delicious and Nutritious Meals for Your Unique Needs

Dr Lily Morgan

COPYRIGHT PAGE

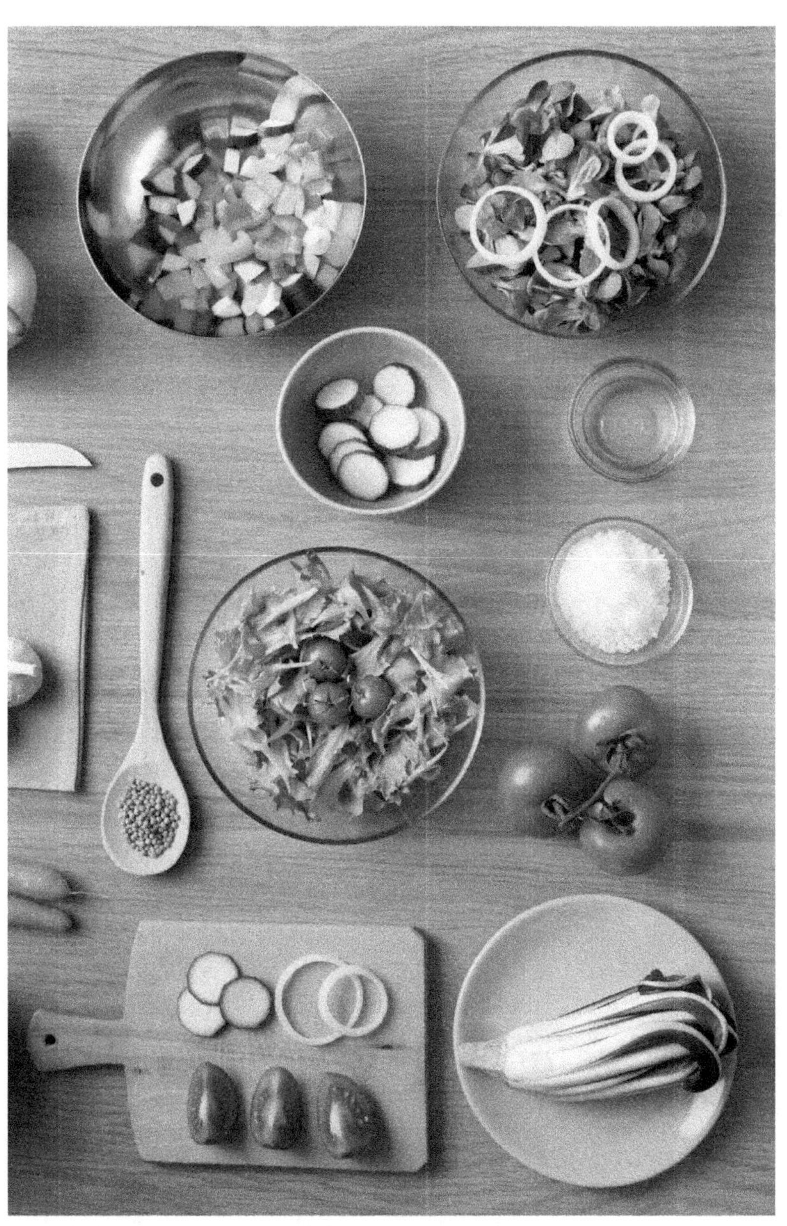

TABLE OF CONTENTS

INTRODUCTION 9

Chapter 1: 30-Day Meal Plan 11

Week 1 11

Week 2 13

Week 3 15

Week 4 18

Chapter 2: Breakfast Recipes 22

Oatmeal with Berries and Almonds 22

Veggie Omelette 23

Whole Grain Pancakes with Sugar-Free Syrup 24

Greek Yogurt Parfait 25

Avocado Toast with Poached Egg 25

Chia Seed Pudding 26

Spinach and Mushroom Frittata 27

Smoothie Bowl 28

Low-Sodium Breakfast Burrito 29

Quinoa Porridge 30

Breakfast Muffins 30

Cinnamon Apple Porridge 31

Sweet Potato Hash 32

Cottage Cheese with Fruit 33

Breakfast Quesadilla 33

Chapter 3: Lunch Recipes.................................. 35

Grilled Chicken Salad....................................... 35

Lentil Soup.. 36

Tuna Salad Lettuce Wraps 37

Quinoa and Black Bean Bowl............................. 37

Turkey and Veggie Wrap................................... 38

Chickpea and Spinach Curry 39

Baked Salmon with Lemon................................ 40

Caprese Salad... 40

Spinach and Strawberry Salad 41

Turkey and Sweet Potato Chili 42

Ratatouille 43

Shrimp Stir-Fry 43

Beef and Broccoli 44

Egg Salad Lettuce Wraps.................................. 45

Mediterranean Chicken Bowl 46

Chapter 4: Dinner Recipes 47

Grilled Portobello Mushrooms 47

Baked Cod with Asparagus................................ 48

Spaghetti Squash Primavera 49

Lemon Herb Roasted Chicken............................. 50

Butternut Squash Soup..................................... 51

Turkey Stuffed Peppers..................................... 52

Sweet and Sour Tofu 52

Pork Tenderloin with Green Beans 53

Eggplant Parmesan 54

Quinoa-Stuffed Bell Peppers 55

Baked Zucchini Boats 56

Beef and Vegetable Stir-Fry 57

Lemon Dill Tilapia 58

Chicken and Broccoli Alfredo 59

Blackened Shrimp 60

Chapter 5: Snacks and Appetizers 61

Guacamole with Veggie Sticks 61

Hummus with Whole Wheat Pita 62

Cucumber and Cottage Cheese Bites 63

Almond-Crusted Chicken Tenders 64

Baked Sweet Potato Fries 65

Deviled Eggs 65

Roasted Red Pepper Dip 66

Greek Salad Skewers 67

Baked Parmesan Zucchini Chips 68

Sliced Apples with Almond Butter 68

Greek Yogurt Dip with Veggies 69

Avocado and Salsa 69

Mixed Nuts 70

Edamame 70

Caprese Skewers 71

Chapter 6: Desserts 72

Sugar-Free Jello with Berries...................................... 72

Baked Apples with Cinnamon 73

Greek Yogurt with Honey and Nuts 73

Chocolate Avocado Mousse 74

Banana Ice Cream 75

Rice Pudding with Raisins 75

Chia Seed Chocolate Pudding...................................... 76

Berry Parfait.. 76

Angel Food Cake with Berries...................................... 77

Frozen Yogurt Popsicles 78

Pumpkin Pie Smoothie... 78

Oatmeal Raisin Cookies.. 79

Carrot Cake Muffins 79

Cinnamon Baked Pears 80

Blueberry Crisp.. 81

Chapter 7: Smoothies 82

Green Power Smoothie 82

Berry Blast Smoothie... 83

Tropical Paradise Smoothie 83

Cucumber and Spinach Smoothie.................................. 84

Avocado and Kale Smoothie 85

Mango Tango Smoothie... 86

Blueberry Almond Smoothie 87

Chocolate Peanut Butter Smoothie 87

Coffee Protein Smoothie... 88

Watermelon Mint Smoothie.. 89

Banana Nut Smoothie 90

Strawberry Kiwi Smoothie 90

Orange Creamsicle Smoothie 91

Spinach and Pineapple Smoothie.. 92

Papaya Passion Smoothie 92

CONCLUSION 94

INTRODUCTION

When it comes to our health, a vital aspect that often goes overlooked is the intricate relationship between kidney health and diabetes. Our kidneys, those bean-shaped organs nestled deep within our bodies, play a pivotal role in maintaining balance. They are the body's filtration system, responsible for cleaning the blood and removing waste products.

Now, why is understanding this connection between kidney health and diabetes so crucial? Diabetes, a condition that affects how our bodies process glucose, can have profound consequences for our kidneys. When blood sugar levels are persistently high, the kidneys are forced to work overtime. Over time, this can lead to damage, reducing their ability to function efficiently.

The Importance of a Kidney-Friendly Diet
The good news is that there are measures we can take to protect our kidney health, particularly if we're dealing with

diabetes. One of the most impactful steps is embracing a kidney-friendly diet. This isn't just about what we eat but also about understanding how specific nutrients and food choices affect our kidneys.

A kidney-friendly diet focuses on maintaining healthy blood pressure and blood sugar levels while minimizing the strain on these essential organs. It typically includes foods that are low in sodium, potassium, and phosphorus. These dietary choices can help in managing diabetes more effectively and reducing the risk of complications, including kidney disease.

So, as we delve into the fascinating world of kidney health and diabetes, we'll explore the science behind these connections, uncover practical dietary recommendations, and ultimately empower ourselves with the knowledge needed to safeguard our health. After all, understanding the intricate interplay of our bodies and making informed choices can lead us on a path to healthier, happier lives.

Chapter 1: 30-Day Meal Plan

Week 1

Day 1:

- Breakfast: Oatmeal with Berries and Almonds
- Lunch: Grilled Chicken Salad
- Dinner: Grilled Portobello Mushrooms
- Snacks: Guacamole with Veggie Sticks
- Dessert: Sugar-Free Jello with Berries

Day 2:

- Breakfast: Veggie Omelette
- Lunch: Lentil Soup
- Dinner: Baked Cod with Asparagus
- Snacks: Hummus with Whole Wheat Pita
- Dessert: Baked Apples with Cinnamon

Day 3:

- Breakfast: Whole Grain Pancakes with Sugar-Free Syrup
- Lunch: Tuna Salad Lettuce Wraps

- Dinner: Spaghetti Squash Primavera
- Snacks: Cucumber and Cottage Cheese Bites
- Dessert: Greek Yogurt with Honey and Nuts

Day 4:

- Breakfast: Greek Yogurt Parfait
- Lunch: Quinoa and Black Bean Bowl
- Dinner: Lemon Herb Roasted Chicken
- Snacks: Almond-Crusted Chicken Tenders
- Dessert: Chocolate Avocado Mousse

Day 5:

- Breakfast: Avocado Toast with Poached Egg
- Lunch: Turkey and Veggie Wrap
- Dinner: Butternut Squash Soup
- Snacks: Baked Sweet Potato Fries
- Dessert: Banana Ice Cream

Day 6:

- Breakfast: Chia Seed Pudding
- Lunch: Chickpea and Spinach Curry
- Dinner: Turkey Stuffed Peppers

- Snacks: Deviled Eggs
- Dessert: Rice Pudding with Raisins

Day 7:

- Breakfast: Spinach and Mushroom Frittata
- Lunch: Baked Salmon with Lemon
- Dinner: Sweet and Sour Tofu
- Snacks: Roasted Red Pepper Dip
- Dessert: Chia Seed Chocolate Pudding

Week 2

Day 8:

- Breakfast: Smoothie Bowl
- Lunch: Caprese Salad
- Dinner: Pork Tenderloin with Green Beans
- Snacks: Greek Salad Skewers
- Dessert: Berry Parfait

Day 9:

- Breakfast: Low-Sodium Breakfast Burrito
- Lunch: Spinach and Strawberry Salad
- Dinner: Eggplant Parmesan

- Snacks: Baked Parmesan Zucchini Chips
- Dessert: Angel Food Cake with Berries

Day 10:

- Breakfast: Quinoa Porridge
- Lunch: Turkey and Sweet Potato Chili
- Dinner: Quinoa-Stuffed Bell Peppers
- Snacks: Sliced Apples with Almond Butter
- Dessert: Frozen Yogurt Popsicles

Day 11:

- Breakfast: Breakfast Muffins
- Lunch: Ratatouille
- Dinner: Baked Zucchini Boats
- Snacks: Greek Yogurt Dip with Veggies
- Dessert: Pumpkin Pie Smoothie

Day 12:

- Breakfast: Cinnamon Apple Porridge
- Lunch: Shrimp Stir-Fry
- Dinner: Beef and Vegetable Stir-Fry
- Snacks: Avocado and Salsa

- Dessert: Oatmeal Raisin Cookies

Day 13:

- Breakfast: Sweet Potato Hash
- Lunch: Beef and Broccoli
- Dinner: Lemon Dill Tilapia
- Snacks: Mixed Nuts
- Dessert: Carrot Cake Muffins

Day 14:

- Breakfast: Cottage Cheese with Fruit
- Lunch: Egg Salad Lettuce Wraps
- Dinner: Chicken and Broccoli Alfredo
- Snacks: Edamame
- Dessert: Cinnamon Baked Pears

Week 3

Day 15:

- Breakfast: Blueberry Crisp
- Lunch: Mediterranean Chicken Bowl
- Dinner: Blackened Shrimp
- Snacks: Caprese Skewers

- Dessert: Sugar-Free Jello with Berries

Day 16:

- Breakfast: Oatmeal with Berries and Almonds
- Lunch: Grilled Chicken Salad
- Dinner: Grilled Portobello Mushrooms
- Snacks: Guacamole with Veggie Sticks
- Dessert: Baked Apples with Cinnamon

Day 17:

- Breakfast: Veggie Omelette
- Lunch: Lentil Soup
- Dinner: Baked Cod with Asparagus
- Snacks: Hummus with Whole Wheat Pita
- Dessert: Greek Yogurt with Honey and Nuts

Day 18:

- Breakfast: Whole Grain Pancakes with Sugar-Free Syrup
- Lunch: Tuna Salad Lettuce Wraps
- Dinner: Spaghetti Squash Primavera
- Snacks: Cucumber and Cottage Cheese Bites

- Dessert: Chocolate Avocado Mousse

Day 19:

- Breakfast: Greek Yogurt Parfait
- Lunch: Quinoa and Black Bean Bowl
- Dinner: Lemon Herb Roasted Chicken
- Snacks: Almond-Crusted Chicken Tenders
- Dessert: Banana Ice Cream

Day 20:

- Breakfast: Avocado Toast with Poached Egg
- Lunch: Turkey and Veggie Wrap
- Dinner: Butternut Squash Soup
- Snacks: Baked Sweet Potato Fries
- Dessert: Rice Pudding with Raisins

Day 21:

- Breakfast: Chia Seed Pudding
- Lunch: Chickpea and Spinach Curry
- Dinner: Turkey Stuffed Peppers
- Snacks: Deviled Eggs
- Dessert: Chia Seed Chocolate Pudding

Week 4

Day 22:

- Breakfast: Sweet Potato Hash
- Lunch: Beef and Broccoli
- Dinner: Lemon Dill Tilapia
- Snacks: Mixed Nuts
- Dessert: Carrot Cake Muffins

Day 23:

- Breakfast: Cottage Cheese with Fruit
- Lunch: Egg Salad Lettuce Wraps
- Dinner: Chicken and Broccoli Alfredo
- Snacks: Edamame
- Dessert: Cinnamon Baked Pears

Day 24:

- Breakfast: Breakfast Quesadilla
- Lunch: Mediterranean Chicken Bowl
- Dinner: Blackened Shrimp
- Snacks: Caprese Skewers
- Dessert: Sugar-Free Jello with Berries

Day 25:

- Breakfast: Oatmeal with Berries and Almonds
- Lunch: Grilled Chicken Salad
- Dinner: Grilled Portobello Mushrooms
- Snacks: Guacamole with Veggie Sticks
- Dessert: Baked Apples with Cinnamon

Day 26:

- Breakfast: Veggie Omelette
- Lunch: Lentil Soup
- Dinner: Baked Cod with Asparagus
- Snacks: Hummus with Whole Wheat Pita
- Dessert: Greek Yogurt with Honey and Nuts

Day 27:

- Breakfast: Whole Grain Pancakes with Sugar-Free Syrup
- Lunch: Tuna Salad Lettuce Wraps
- Dinner: Spaghetti Squash Primavera
- Snacks: Cucumber and Cottage Cheese Bites
- Dessert: Chocolate Avocado Mousse

Day 28:

- Breakfast: Greek Yogurt Parfait
- Lunch: Quinoa and Black Bean Bowl
- Dinner: Lemon Herb Roasted Chicken
- Snacks: Almond-Crusted Chicken Tenders
- Dessert: Banana Ice Cream

Day 29:

- Breakfast: Avocado Toast with Poached Egg
- Lunch: Turkey and Veggie Wrap
- Dinner: Butternut Squash Soup
- Snacks: Baked Sweet Potato Fries
- Dessert: Rice Pudding with Raisins

Day 30:

- Breakfast: Chia Seed Pudding
- Lunch: Chickpea and Spinach Curry
- Dinner: Turkey Stuffed Peppers
- Snacks: Deviled Eggs
- Dessert: Chia Seed Chocolate Pudding

This completes the 30-day meal plan with a variety of kidney-friendly diabetic recipes for each day. Enjoy your delicious and health-conscious meals while managing your health.

Chapter 2: Breakfast Recipes

Start your day with a nutritious and delicious breakfast that's both kidney-friendly and suitable for those managing diabetes. These breakfast recipes are thoughtfully crafted to provide you with a variety of flavors and options to keep your mornings exciting. Each recipe is packed with essential nutrients and flavors that will help you kickstart your day with a burst of energy.

Oatmeal with Berries and Almonds

Ingredients:

- 1/2 cup rolled oats
- 1 cup unsweetened almond milk
- 1/4 cup fresh berries (e.g., blueberries, strawberries)
- 1 tablespoon chopped almonds
- 1 teaspoon honey or a sugar substitute (optional)

Instructions:

1. In a saucepan, combine the oats and almond milk.

2. Cook over medium heat, stirring frequently, until the oatmeal reaches your desired consistency.

3. Transfer the oatmeal to a bowl and top it with fresh berries and chopped almonds.

4. Drizzle with a touch of honey if you prefer a sweeter taste.

Veggie Omelette

Ingredients:

- 2 large eggs
- 1/4 cup diced bell peppers (any color)
- 1/4 cup diced onions
- 1/4 cup diced tomatoes
- Salt and pepper to taste
- Cooking spray or a small amount of olive oil

Instructions:

1. In a bowl, beat the eggs and season with salt and pepper.

2. Heat a non-stick skillet over medium-high heat and lightly grease with cooking spray or olive oil.

3. Add the diced vegetables to the skillet and sauté until they become tender.

4. Pour the beaten eggs over the veggies and cook until the edges are set.

5. Carefully fold the omelette in half and continue cooking until the center is fully cooked.

Whole Grain Pancakes with Sugar-Free Syrup

Ingredients:

- 1/2 cup whole grain pancake mix
- 1/2 cup water or unsweetened almond milk
- Sugar-free pancake syrup

Instructions:

1. Prepare the pancake mix according to the package instructions, using water or almond milk.

2. Heat a griddle or non-stick pan over medium heat and lightly grease it.

3. Pour the pancake batter onto the griddle to create the desired pancake size.

4. Cook until bubbles form on the surface, then flip and cook until golden brown.

5. Serve with sugar-free pancake syrup.

Greek Yogurt Parfait

Ingredients:

- 1/2 cup plain Greek yogurt
- 1/4 cup fresh berries
- 1 tablespoon honey or sugar substitute (optional)
- 2 tablespoons granola

Instructions:

1. In a glass or bowl, layer the Greek yogurt, fresh berries, and granola.
2. Drizzle with honey if desired.

Avocado Toast with Poached Egg

Ingredients:

- 1 slice whole-grain bread
- 1/2 ripe avocado, mashed
- 1 poached egg

- Salt and pepper to taste
- Optional toppings: sliced tomatoes, red pepper flakes, or a sprinkle of feta cheese

Instructions:

1. Toast the bread to your desired level of crispness.
2. Spread the mashed avocado on the toasted bread.
3. Top with a poached egg and season with salt and pepper.
4. Add optional toppings if desired.

Chia Seed Pudding

Ingredients:

- 2 tablespoons chia seeds
- 1/2 cup unsweetened almond milk
- 1/2 teaspoon vanilla extract
- 1/2 cup fresh berries
- 1 teaspoon honey or sugar substitute (optional)

Instructions:

1. In a jar or bowl, mix the chia seeds, almond milk, and vanilla extract.

2. Stir well, cover, and refrigerate overnight or for at least a few hours to allow the chia seeds to absorb the liquid and thicken.

3. Serve with fresh berries and a drizzle of honey if desired.

Spinach and Mushroom Frittata

Ingredients:

- 4 large eggs
- 1 cup fresh spinach, chopped
- 1/2 cup mushrooms, sliced
- 1/4 cup diced onions
- Salt and pepper to taste
- Cooking spray or a small amount of olive oil

Instructions:

1. Preheat the oven to 350°F (175°C).
2. In a bowl, beat the eggs and season with salt and pepper.
3. Heat an oven-safe skillet over medium-high heat and lightly grease with cooking spray or olive oil.
4. Sauté the onions and mushrooms until they soften.

5. Add the chopped spinach and cook until wilted.

6. Pour the beaten eggs over the vegetables and cook for a minute without stirring.

7. Transfer the skillet to the preheated oven and bake for about 10-15 minutes or until the frittata is set and slightly golden.

Smoothie Bowl

Ingredients:

- 1 cup unsweetened almond milk
- 1/2 cup frozen mixed berries
- 1/2 banana
- 1 tablespoon almond butter
- Toppings: sliced banana, fresh berries, granola, and a drizzle of honey (optional)

Instructions:

1. Blend the almond milk, mixed berries, banana, and almond butter until smooth.

2. Pour the smoothie into a bowl and add your choice of toppings.

Low-Sodium Breakfast Burrito

Ingredients:

- 2 large eggs
- 1/4 cup diced bell peppers (any color)
- 1/4 cup diced onions
- 1/4 cup diced tomatoes
- 1 whole wheat tortilla
- Salt and pepper to taste

Instructions:

1. In a bowl, beat the eggs and season with salt and pepper.
2. Heat a non-stick skillet over medium-high heat.
3. Add the diced vegetables to the skillet and sauté until they become tender.
4. Pour the beaten eggs over the veggies and cook until they are fully scrambled.
5. Warm the tortilla and place the scrambled eggs in the center.
6. Fold the sides of the tortilla and roll it up to create a burrito.

Quinoa Porridge

Ingredients:

- 1/2 cup cooked quinoa
- 1/2 cup unsweetened almond milk
- 1/4 cup fresh berries
- 1 teaspoon honey or sugar substitute (optional)

Instructions:

1. In a saucepan, combine the cooked quinoa and almond milk.
2. Cook over medium heat, stirring frequently, until the porridge reaches your desired consistency.
3. Serve with fresh berries and a drizzle of honey if desired.

Breakfast Muffins

Ingredients:

- 2 eggs
- 1/4 cup diced bell peppers (any color)
- 1/4 cup diced onions
- 1/4 cup diced tomatoes

- Salt and pepper to taste
- Cooking spray

Instructions:

1. Preheat the oven to 350°F (175°C).
2. In a bowl, beat the eggs and season with salt and pepper.
3. Grease a muffin tin with cooking spray.
4. Divide the diced vegetables evenly among the muffin cups.
5. Pour the beaten eggs over the vegetables.
6. Bake for about 15-20 minutes or until the muffins are set and slightly golden.

Cinnamon Apple Porridge

Ingredients:

- 1/2 cup rolled oats
- 1 cup unsweetened almond milk
- 1/2 apple, diced
- 1/2 teaspoon ground cinnamon
- 1 teaspoon honey or sugar substitute (optional)

Instructions:

1. In a saucepan, combine the oats, almond milk, diced apple, and ground cinnamon.
2. Cook over medium heat, stirring frequently, until the porridge reaches your desired consistency.
3. Drizzle with honey if you prefer a sweeter taste.

Sweet Potato Hash

Ingredients:

- 1 small sweet potato, peeled and diced
- 1/4 cup diced onions
- 1/4 cup diced bell peppers (any color)
- 1/4 cup diced tomatoes
- 1/4 teaspoon paprika
- Salt and pepper to taste
- Cooking spray or a small amount of olive oil

Instructions:

1. Heat a skillet over medium heat and lightly grease with cooking spray or olive oil.
2. Add the diced sweet potatoes and sauté until they are tender and slightly crispy.

3. Add the onions, bell peppers, and tomatoes and cook until they are softened.

4. Season with paprika, salt, and pepper.

Cottage Cheese with Fruit

Ingredients:

- 1/2 cup low-fat cottage cheese
- 1/2 cup fresh fruit (e.g., sliced peaches, pineapple, or berries)
- 1 teaspoon honey or sugar substitute (optional)

Instructions:

1. In a bowl, layer the cottage cheese and fresh fruit.

2. Drizzle with honey if desired.

Breakfast Quesadilla

Ingredients:

- 1 whole wheat tortilla
- 2 large eggs
- 1/4 cup diced bell peppers (any color)
- 1/4 cup diced onions

- 1/4 cup diced tomatoes
- 2 tablespoons shredded low-fat cheese
- Salt and pepper to taste

Instructions:

1. In a bowl, beat the eggs and season with salt and pepper.
2. Heat a non-stick skillet over medium-high heat.
3. Add the diced vegetables to the skillet and sauté until they become tender.
4. Pour the beaten eggs over the veggies and cook until they are fully scrambled.
5. Place the whole wheat tortilla in the skillet and sprinkle it with shredded cheese.
6. Spoon the scrambled eggs and veggies over one half of the tortilla and fold the other half over to create a quesadilla.

Chapter 3: Lunch Recipes

In this chapter, we delve into a variety of satisfying and nutritious lunch options that are not only delicious but also suitable for kidney health and diabetes management. These recipes are designed to provide a balance of flavors and nutrients, ensuring that your midday meal is both enjoyable and supportive of your well-being.

Grilled Chicken Salad

Ingredients:

- Boneless, skinless chicken breast
- Mixed salad greens
- Cherry tomatoes
- Cucumber
- Red onion
- Balsamic vinaigrette

Instructions:

1. Grill the chicken breast until fully cooked.
2. Slice the grilled chicken into thin strips.

3. Toss mixed salad greens, cherry tomatoes, cucumber, and red onion in a bowl.

4. Top the salad with the grilled chicken.

5. Drizzle with balsamic vinaigrette and enjoy!

Lentil Soup

Ingredients:

- Red lentils
- Onion
- Carrots
- Celery
- Vegetable broth
- Cumin
- Paprika
- Salt and pepper

Instructions:

1. Sauté onion, carrots, and celery in a pot until tender.

2. Add red lentils, vegetable broth, cumin, and paprika.

3. Simmer until the lentils are soft.

4. Season with salt and pepper.

5. Serve hot.

Tuna Salad Lettuce Wraps

Ingredients:

- Canned tuna in water
- Greek yogurt
- Dijon mustard
- Celery
- Red onion
- Lettuce leaves

Instructions:

1. Mix tuna, Greek yogurt, Dijon mustard, celery, and red onion.
2. Spoon the tuna salad into lettuce leaves.
3. Roll them up and enjoy this low-carb option.

Quinoa and Black Bean Bowl

Ingredients:

- Cooked quinoa
- Black beans
- Corn
- Bell peppers

- Avocado

- Lime juice

- Cilantro

Instructions:

1. Combine quinoa, black beans, corn, and diced bell peppers.

2. Top with sliced avocado.

3. Drizzle with lime juice and garnish with cilantro.

Turkey and Veggie Wrap

Ingredients:

- Whole wheat tortilla

- Sliced turkey breast

- Hummus

- Baby spinach

- Sliced cucumber

- Sliced bell peppers

Instructions:

1. Spread hummus on the tortilla.

2. Layer turkey, spinach, cucumber, and bell peppers.

3. Roll it up, slice, and serve.

Chickpea and Spinach Curry

Ingredients:

- Chickpeas
- Spinach
- Onion
- Garlic
- Tomatoes
- Curry powder
- Coconut milk

Instructions:

1. Sauté chopped onion and garlic in a pot.
2. Add curry powder and cook for a minute.
3. Stir in chickpeas, chopped tomatoes, and coconut milk.
4. Simmer until the sauce thickens.
5. Add spinach and cook until wilted.

Baked Salmon with Lemon

Ingredients:

- Salmon fillet
- Lemon juice
- Dill
- Garlic
- Olive oil
- Salt and pepper

Instructions:

1. Preheat the oven to 350°F (175°C).
2. Place salmon on a baking sheet.
3. Drizzle with lemon juice and olive oil.
4. Season with dill, garlic, salt, and pepper.
5. Bake for about 15-20 minutes or until the salmon flakes easily.

Caprese Salad

Ingredients:

- Tomatoes
- Fresh mozzarella

- Fresh basil leaves

- Balsamic vinegar

- Olive oil

- Salt and pepper

Instructions:

1. Slice tomatoes and fresh mozzarella.

2. Arrange them with basil leaves on a plate.

3. Drizzle with balsamic vinegar and olive oil.

4. Season with salt and pepper.

Spinach and Strawberry Salad

Ingredients:

- Baby spinach

- Sliced strawberries

- Almonds

- Feta cheese

- Balsamic vinaigrette

Instructions:

1. Combine baby spinach, sliced strawberries, and almonds in a bowl.

2. Crumble feta cheese on top.

3. Drizzle with balsamic vinaigrette.

Turkey and Sweet Potato Chili

Ingredients:

- Ground turkey
- Sweet potatoes
- Kidney beans
- Tomatoes
- Chili powder
- Cumin
- Paprika

Instructions:

1. Brown ground turkey in a pot.

2. Add diced sweet potatoes, kidney beans, and canned tomatoes.

3. Season with chili powder, cumin, and paprika.

4. Simmer until sweet potatoes are tender.

Ratatouille

Ingredients:

- Eggplant
- Zucchini
- Bell peppers
- Onion
- Tomatoes
- Garlic
- Herbs (thyme, basil, oregano)
- Olive oil

Instructions:

1. Sauté chopped onion and garlic in a large skillet.
2. Layer sliced eggplant, zucchini, bell peppers, and tomatoes.
3. Season with herbs and drizzle with olive oil.
4. Cover and cook until the veggies are tender.

Shrimp Stir-Fry

Ingredients:

- Shrimp

- Mixed vegetables (broccoli, bell peppers, snap peas)
- Garlic
- Ginger
- Soy sauce
- Sesame oil

Instructions:

1. Sauté minced garlic and ginger in a wok.
2. Add shrimp and stir-fry until pink.
3. Add mixed vegetables, soy sauce, and sesame oil.
4. Cook until the veggies are crisp-tender.

Beef and Broccoli

Ingredients:

- Thinly sliced beef
- Broccoli florets
- Garlic
- Soy sauce
- Brown sugar
- Ginger
- Cornstarch

Instructions:

1. Mix soy sauce, brown sugar, ginger, and cornstarch in a bowl.
2. Sauté garlic and beef in a skillet.
3. Add broccoli and the sauce mixture.
4. Cook until the sauce thickens.

Egg Salad Lettuce Wraps

Ingredients:

- Hard-boiled eggs
- Greek yogurt
- Dijon mustard
- Celery
- Green onions
- Lettuce leaves

Instructions:

1. Chop hard-boiled eggs and mix with Greek yogurt, Dijon mustard, celery, and green onions.
2. Spoon the egg salad into lettuce leaves.
3. Roll them up for a light and satisfying meal.

Mediterranean Chicken Bowl

Ingredients:

- Grilled chicken breast
- Quinoa
- Cherry tomatoes
- Cucumber
- Kalamata olives
- Feta cheese
- Tzatziki sauce

Instructions:

1. Slice grilled chicken and arrange it in a bowl.

2. Add cooked quinoa, halved cherry tomatoes, sliced cucumber, Kalamata olives, and crumbled feta cheese.

3. Drizzle with tzatziki sauce for a Mediterranean delight.

Chapter 4: Dinner Recipes

In this chapter, we explore a delightful array of dinner recipes that are not only kidney-friendly but also perfect for those managing diabetes. These dishes are designed to tantalize your taste buds while keeping your health in mind. Let's dive into these delicious and nutritious dinner options.

Grilled Portobello Mushrooms

Ingredients:

- 4 large portobello mushrooms
- 2 tablespoons olive oil
- 2 cloves garlic, minced
- 1 teaspoon balsamic vinegar
- Salt and pepper to taste

Instructions:

1. Preheat the grill to medium-high heat.
2. Clean the mushrooms and remove the stems.
3. In a small bowl, mix olive oil, minced garlic, balsamic vinegar, salt, and pepper.

4. Brush the mushroom caps with the mixture.

5. Grill the mushrooms for about 5 minutes on each side until tender.

Baked Cod with Asparagus

Ingredients:

- 4 cod fillets
- 1 bunch asparagus
- 2 tablespoons olive oil
- 1 lemon, sliced
- Salt and pepper to taste

Instructions:

1. Preheat the oven to 375°F (190°C).
2. Place the cod fillets on a baking sheet.
3. Arrange asparagus around the fish.
4. Drizzle olive oil over the fish and asparagus.
5. Season with salt and pepper.
6. Top with lemon slices.
7. Bake for 15-20 minutes until the cod is flaky and asparagus is tender.

Spaghetti Squash Primavera

Ingredients:

- 1 spaghetti squash
- 2 cups mixed vegetables (e.g., bell peppers, broccoli, carrots)
- 2 tablespoons olive oil
- 2 cloves garlic, minced
- 1 cup cherry tomatoes, halved
- Fresh basil leaves
- Grated Parmesan cheese (optional)

Instructions:

1. Preheat the oven to 375°F (190°C).
2. Cut the spaghetti squash in half lengthwise and remove the seeds.
3. Drizzle with olive oil, season with salt and pepper, and place face down on a baking sheet.
4. Roast for 30-40 minutes until the squash is tender.
5. While the squash is roasting, sauté mixed vegetables and garlic in a pan until tender.
6. Scrape the cooked spaghetti squash with a fork to create "noodles."

7. Toss the squash with sautéed vegetables and cherry tomatoes.

8. Garnish with fresh basil leaves and Parmesan cheese if desired.

Lemon Herb Roasted Chicken

Ingredients:

- 4 boneless, skinless chicken breasts
- 2 tablespoons olive oil
- 2 cloves garlic, minced
- Zest and juice of 1 lemon
- 1 teaspoon dried thyme
- Salt and pepper to taste

Instructions:

1. Preheat the oven to 375°F (190°C).

2. In a bowl, mix olive oil, garlic, lemon zest, lemon juice, dried thyme, salt, and pepper.

3. Place chicken breasts in a baking dish and brush with the lemon herb mixture.

4. Roast for about 25-30 minutes until the chicken is cooked through.

Butternut Squash Soup

Ingredients:

- 1 butternut squash, peeled, seeded, and cubed
- 1 onion, chopped
- 2 cloves garlic, minced
- 1 carrot, chopped
- 4 cups low-sodium chicken or vegetable broth
- 1 teaspoon dried sage
- Salt and pepper to taste

Instructions:

1. In a large pot, sauté onion, garlic, and carrot until soft.
2. Add butternut squash, broth, dried sage, salt, and pepper.
3. Bring to a boil, then reduce heat and simmer for 20-25 minutes.
4. Blend until smooth using an immersion blender or countertop blender.
5. Return to the pot and heat through before serving.

Turkey Stuffed Peppers

Ingredients:

- 4 bell peppers
- 1 pound ground turkey
- 1 cup cooked quinoa
- 1 can low-sodium diced tomatoes
- 1 teaspoon Italian seasoning
- Salt and pepper to taste

Instructions:

1. Preheat the oven to 375°F (190°C).
2. Cut the tops off the bell peppers and remove seeds.
3. In a bowl, mix ground turkey, cooked quinoa, diced tomatoes, Italian seasoning, salt, and pepper.
4. Stuff each bell pepper with the turkey mixture.
5. Place in a baking dish and bake for 30-40 minutes until peppers are tender.

Sweet and Sour Tofu

Ingredients:

- 1 block extra-firm tofu, cubed

- 1 bell pepper, sliced

- 1 cup pineapple chunks

- 1/4 cup low-sodium soy sauce

- 2 tablespoons rice vinegar

- 2 tablespoons brown sugar

- 1 tablespoon cornstarch

- 1/4 cup water

- Sesame seeds for garnish (optional)

Instructions:

1. In a bowl, whisk together soy sauce, rice vinegar, brown sugar, cornstarch, and water.
2. Heat a pan and add tofu, bell pepper, and pineapple.
3. Pour the sweet and sour sauce over the tofu mixture.
4. Cook until the sauce thickens and everything is heated through.
5. Garnish with sesame seeds if desired.

Pork Tenderloin with Green Beans

Ingredients:

- 1 pork tenderloin

- 1 pound green beans

- 2 tablespoons olive oil

- 2 cloves garlic, minced

- 1 teaspoon dried rosemary

- Salt and pepper to taste

Instructions:

1. Preheat the oven to 375°F (190°C).

2. Season the pork tenderloin with salt, pepper, and dried rosemary.

3. In a large ovenproof skillet, heat olive oil over medium-high heat.

4. Sear the pork on all sides until browned.

5. Add green beans and minced garlic to the skillet.

6. Roast in the oven for 20-25 minutes until the pork is cooked through and the beans are tender.

Eggplant Parmesan

Ingredients:

- 2 large eggplants, sliced

- 1 cup marinara sauce

- 1 cup part-skim mozzarella cheese, shredded

- 1/4 cup grated Parmesan cheese

- 1/4 cup fresh basil leaves
- Olive oil for frying

Instructions:

1. Heat olive oil in a pan over medium heat.
2. Fry the eggplant slices until they are golden brown.
3. Preheat the oven to 375°F (190°C).
4. In a baking dish, layer eggplant, marinara sauce, mozzarella, and Parmesan cheese.
5. Repeat the layers and top with fresh basil leaves.
6. Bake for 25-30 minutes until the cheese is bubbly and golden.

Quinoa-Stuffed Bell Peppers

Ingredients:

- 4 bell peppers
- 1 cup cooked quinoa
- 1 can low-sodium black beans, drained and rinsed
- 1 cup corn kernels
- 1 cup diced tomatoes
- 1 teaspoon chili powder
- Salt and pepper to taste

Instructions:

1. Preheat the oven to 375°F (190°C).

2. Cut the tops off the bell peppers and remove seeds.

3. In a bowl, mix cooked quinoa, black beans, corn, diced tomatoes, chili powder, salt, and pepper.

4. Stuff each bell pepper with the quinoa mixture.

5. Place in a baking dish and bake for 30-40 minutes until peppers are tender.

Baked Zucchini Boats

Ingredients:

*   4 zucchinis

*   1 pound lean ground beef or turkey

*   1 cup low-sodium marinara sauce

*   1 cup part-skim mozzarella cheese, shredded

*   1/4 cup chopped fresh basil

*   Salt and pepper to taste

Instructions:

1. Preheat the oven to 375°F (190°C).

2. Slice zucchinis in half lengthwise and scoop out the centers to create "boats."

3. In a skillet, brown the ground meat, drain excess fat.

4. Mix in marinara sauce, salt, and pepper.

5. Fill the zucchini boats with the meat mixture.

6. Sprinkle mozzarella cheese on top.

7. Bake for 25-30 minutes until zucchinis are tender.

Beef and Vegetable Stir-Fry

Ingredients:

- 1 pound lean beef, thinly sliced
- 2 cups mixed vegetables (e.g., broccoli, bell peppers, carrots)
- 2 tablespoons low-sodium soy sauce
- 1 tablespoon honey
- 1 teaspoon ginger, minced
- 2 cloves garlic, minced
- 1 tablespoon cornstarch
- Cooked brown rice (optional)

Instructions:

1. In a small bowl, mix soy sauce, honey, ginger, garlic, and cornstarch.

2. Heat a large skillet over high heat.

3. Stir-fry the beef until browned and set aside.

4. Add mixed vegetables to the skillet and stir-fry until tender.

5. Return the beef to the skillet and pour the sauce over it.

6. Cook until the sauce thickens.

7. Serve over cooked brown rice if desired.

Lemon Dill Tilapia

Ingredients:

- 4 tilapia fillets
- Zest and juice of 1 lemon
- 2 tablespoons olive oil
- 1 teaspoon dried dill
- Salt and pepper to taste

Instructions:

1. Preheat the oven to 375°F (190°C).

2. In a bowl, mix lemon zest, lemon juice, olive oil, dried dill, salt, and pepper.

3. Place tilapia fillets on a baking sheet and brush with the lemon mixture.

4. Bake for about 15-20 minutes until the fish flakes
    easily.

Chicken and Broccoli Alfredo

Ingredients:

- 2 boneless, skinless chicken breasts
- 2 cups broccoli florets
- 8 oz whole wheat pasta
- 1 cup low-fat Alfredo sauce
- Salt and pepper to taste
- Grated Parmesan cheese for garnish (optional)

Instructions:

1. Cook the pasta according to package instructions.
2. Season chicken with salt and pepper, then grill or
    cook in a pan until done.
3. Steam broccoli until tender.
4. Slice cooked chicken into strips.
5. In a large skillet, mix cooked pasta, chicken,
    broccoli, and Alfredo sauce.
6. Heat through and garnish with Parmesan cheese if
    desired.

Blackened Shrimp

Ingredients:

- 1 pound large shrimp, peeled and deveined
- 1 tablespoon olive oil
- 1 tablespoon blackened seasoning
- 1 lemon, sliced
- Fresh parsley for garnish

Instructions:

1. In a bowl, toss shrimp with olive oil and blackened seasoning.
2. Heat a skillet over medium-high heat.
3. Cook shrimp for 2-3 minutes on each side until they turn pink and slightly crispy.
4. Serve with lemon slices and garnish with fresh parsley.

Chapter 5: Snacks and Appetizers

When it comes to satisfying your cravings between meals or impressing your guests with delectable appetizers, this chapter is your ultimate guide. We've handpicked a diverse range of snacks and appetizers that are not only delicious but also suitable for kidney-friendly and diabetic diets.

Guacamole with Veggie Sticks

Ingredients:

- 2 ripe avocados
- 1 small onion, finely chopped
- 1-2 cloves of garlic, minced
- 1 ripe tomato, diced
- 1 lime, juiced
- Salt and pepper to taste
- Carrot sticks, cucumber slices, and bell pepper strips for dipping

Instructions:

1. Cut the avocados in half, remove the pits, and scoop the flesh into a bowl.
2. Mash the avocado with a fork until it reaches your desired consistency.
3. Add the chopped onion, minced garlic, diced tomato, and lime juice. Mix well.
4. Season with salt and pepper to taste.
5. Serve with veggie sticks for a nutritious and satisfying snack.

Hummus with Whole Wheat Pita

Ingredients:

- 1 can (15 oz) of chickpeas, drained and rinsed
- 2 cloves of garlic
- 3 tablespoons of tahini
- 3 tablespoons of lemon juice
- 2 tablespoons of olive oil
- Salt and cumin to taste
- Whole wheat pita bread, cut into triangles

Instructions:

1. In a food processor, blend the chickpeas, garlic, tahini, lemon juice, and olive oil until smooth.

2. Season with salt and cumin to taste.

3. Serve the hummus with whole wheat pita triangles for a delightful dip.

Cucumber and Cottage Cheese Bites

Ingredients:

- 1 cucumber, sliced into rounds
- Low-fat cottage cheese
- Fresh dill or chives for garnish

Instructions:

1. Place a dollop of low-fat cottage cheese on each cucumber slice.

2. Garnish with fresh dill or chives.

3. Enjoy these refreshing and creamy bites.

Almond-Crusted Chicken Tenders

Ingredients:

- 1 lb chicken tenders
- 1 cup almond meal
- 1 teaspoon paprika
- 1/2 teaspoon garlic powder
- Salt and pepper to taste
- Olive oil for baking

Instructions:

1. Preheat your oven to 375°F (190°C).
2. In a bowl, combine almond meal, paprika, garlic powder, salt, and pepper.
3. Dip each chicken tender into the almond mixture, pressing the coating onto the chicken.
4. Place the coated tenders on a baking sheet lined with parchment paper.
5. Drizzle with olive oil and bake for 20-25 minutes or until the chicken is cooked through and the coating is golden.

Baked Sweet Potato Fries

Ingredients:

- 2 sweet potatoes, cut into fries
- 2 tablespoons olive oil
- 1/2 teaspoon paprika
- 1/2 teaspoon garlic powder
- Salt and pepper to taste

Instructions:

1. Preheat your oven to 425°F (220°C).
2. Toss sweet potato fries with olive oil, paprika, garlic powder, salt, and pepper.
3. Spread them on a baking sheet and bake for 20-25 minutes, flipping once, until they're crispy and golden.

Deviled Eggs

Ingredients:

- 6 large eggs, hard-boiled and peeled
- 3 tablespoons mayonnaise
- 1 teaspoon Dijon mustard

- Salt and pepper to taste
- Paprika for garnish

Instructions:

1. Slice the hard-boiled eggs in half lengthwise and remove the yolks.
2. In a bowl, mash the yolks, then mix in mayonnaise, Dijon mustard, salt, and pepper.
3. Fill the egg white halves with the yolk mixture and sprinkle with paprika.

Roasted Red Pepper Dip

Ingredients:

- 2 red bell peppers
- 1/2 cup plain Greek yogurt
- 2 cloves of garlic
- 1 tablespoon olive oil
- Salt and pepper to taste
- Fresh parsley for garnish

Instructions:

1. Roast the red bell peppers until the skin is charred, then peel and deseed them.

2. In a food processor, blend the roasted peppers, garlic, Greek yogurt, olive oil, salt, and pepper until smooth.

3. Garnish with fresh parsley and serve with veggies.

Greek Salad Skewers

Ingredients:

- Cherry tomatoes
- Cucumber chunks
- Feta cheese cubes
- Kalamata olives
- Fresh basil leaves
- Balsamic glaze for drizzling

Instructions:

1. Thread cherry tomatoes, cucumber chunks, feta cheese, Kalamata olives, and fresh basil leaves onto skewers.

2. Drizzle with balsamic glaze for a taste of the Mediterranean.

Baked Parmesan Zucchini Chips

Ingredients:

- 2 medium zucchinis, sliced into thin rounds
- 1/2 cup grated Parmesan cheese
- 1/2 teaspoon garlic powder
- 1/2 teaspoon dried basil
- Olive oil for brushing

Instructions:

1. Preheat your oven to 425°F (220°C).
2. In a bowl, mix the Parmesan cheese, garlic powder, and dried basil.
3. Brush the zucchini slices with olive oil, then coat them in the Parmesan mixture.
4. Place the coated zucchini rounds on a baking sheet and bake for about 20 minutes or until they're golden and crispy.

Sliced Apples with Almond Butter

Ingredients:

- Apples, thinly sliced

- Almond butter for dipping

Instructions:

1. Simply slice some fresh apples and serve them with almond butter for a wholesome and satisfying snack.

Greek Yogurt Dip with Veggies

Ingredients:

- Greek yogurt
- Assorted fresh vegetables for dipping (e.g., carrot sticks, cucumber slices, bell pepper strips)

Instructions:

1. Use Greek yogurt as a creamy dip for your fresh veggies. It's a simple yet nutritious combination that's perfect for snacking.

Avocado and Salsa

Ingredients:

- Ripe avocados
- Fresh salsa

Instructions:

1. Slice ripe avocados and serve them with a side of fresh salsa. This combo is packed with flavor and healthy fats.

Mixed Nuts

Ingredients:

- An assortment of mixed nuts (unsalted for kidney health)

Instructions:

1. A handful of mixed nuts makes for a quick, satisfying, and heart-healthy snack.

Edamame

Ingredients:

- Edamame beans, steamed and lightly salted

Instructions:

1. Enjoy steamed edamame beans as a nutritious snack. They're rich in protein and fiber.

Caprese Skewers

Ingredients:

- Cherry tomatoes
- Fresh mozzarella balls
- Fresh basil leaves
- Balsamic glaze for drizzling

Instructions:

1. Thread cherry tomatoes, fresh mozzarella, and basil leaves onto skewers, then drizzle with balsamic glaze. These skewers are a delightful burst of flavors.

Chapter 6: Desserts

Desserts are the delightful conclusion to any meal, and when dealing with kidney-friendly diabetic recipes, you can still enjoy sweet treats that are both delicious and healthy. Here, we present 15 dessert recipes that are tailored to your dietary needs. These treats will satisfy your sweet tooth without compromising your health.

Sugar-Free Jello with Berries

Ingredients:

- Sugar-free raspberry Jello mix
- Mixed berries (strawberries, blueberries, raspberries)
- Water

Instructions:

1. Prepare the Jello mix according to the package instructions.
2. Pour the Jello mixture into serving cups and add mixed berries.
3. Refrigerate until set.

4. Serve and enjoy your fruity Jello dessert!

Baked Apples with Cinnamon

Ingredients:

- Apples
- Ground cinnamon
- A touch of brown sugar (or sugar substitute)

Instructions:

1. Preheat your oven to 350°F (175°C).
2. Core the apples, leaving the bottoms intact.
3. Sprinkle cinnamon and a small amount of brown sugar inside each apple.
4. Bake for 30-40 minutes until the apples are soft.
5. Serve warm and savor the warm, fragrant goodness.

Greek Yogurt with Honey and Nuts

Ingredients:

- Greek yogurt
- Honey

- Chopped mixed nuts (almonds, walnuts, or pistachios)

Instructions:

1. Spoon Greek yogurt into serving bowls.
2. Drizzle honey over the yogurt.
3. Sprinkle chopped nuts on top.
4. Dive into the creamy, nutty delight.

Chocolate Avocado Mousse

Ingredients:

- Ripe avocados
- Unsweetened cocoa powder
- Honey or sugar substitute
- Vanilla extract

Instructions:

1. Blend avocados, cocoa powder, honey, and a dash of vanilla extract until smooth.
2. Chill in the refrigerator for an hour.
3. Serve this rich and healthy chocolate mousse.

Banana Ice Cream

Ingredients:

- Ripe bananas
- Vanilla extract
- A pinch of cinnamon

Instructions:

1. Slice bananas and freeze until solid.
2. Blend the frozen bananas, a dash of vanilla extract, and a pinch of cinnamon until creamy.
3. Scoop and relish this natural, sugar-free ice cream.

Rice Pudding with Raisins

Ingredients:

- Brown rice
- Unsweetened almond milk
- Raisins
- Cinnamon

Instructions:

1. Cook brown rice in almond milk until it's creamy.

2. Stir in raisins and a sprinkle of cinnamon.

3. Warm your soul with this comforting rice pudding.

Chia Seed Chocolate Pudding

Ingredients:

- Chia seeds

- Unsweetened almond milk

- Unsweetened cocoa powder

- Honey or sugar substitute

Instructions:

1. Mix chia seeds, almond milk, cocoa powder, and sweetener.

2. Let it sit in the fridge overnight.

3. Satisfy your sweet cravings with this chocolaty delight.

Berry Parfait

Ingredients:

- Mixed berries

- Greek yogurt

- Granola (make sure it's low in sugar)

Instructions:

1. Layer mixed berries, Greek yogurt, and granola in a glass.
2. Repeat the layers.
3. Top with a few more berries for a refreshing parfait.

Angel Food Cake with Berries

Ingredients:

- Store-bought or homemade angel food cake
- Fresh mixed berries
- Whipped cream (sugar-free)

Instructions:

1. Slice the angel food cake into serving portions.
2. Top with mixed berries and a dollop of sugar-free whipped cream.
3. Enjoy a heavenly dessert.

Frozen Yogurt Popsicles

Ingredients:

- Greek yogurt
- Mixed berries
- Honey or sugar substitute

Instructions:

1. Mix Greek yogurt with berries and sweetener.
2. Pour the mixture into popsicle molds and freeze.
3. Savor these cooling popsicles on a warm day.

Pumpkin Pie Smoothie

Ingredients:

- Canned pumpkin puree
- Almond milk
- Cinnamon and nutmeg
- Honey or sugar substitute

Instructions:

1. Blend pumpkin puree, almond milk, spices, and sweetener.

2. Enjoy the flavors of pumpkin pie in a creamy smoothie.

Oatmeal Raisin Cookies

Ingredients:

- Rolled oats
- Raisins
- Cinnamon
- Banana (for natural sweetness)

Instructions:

1. Mash the banana and mix it with oats, raisins, and cinnamon.
2. Form into cookies and bake until golden brown.
3. Relish these guilt-free oatmeal cookies.

Carrot Cake Muffins

Ingredients:

- Grated carrots
- Whole wheat flour
- Chopped nuts

- Cinnamon

Instructions:

1. Combine grated carrots, whole wheat flour, nuts, and cinnamon to make muffin batter.
2. Bake until they're moist and delightful.
3. Enjoy the flavors of carrot cake in muffin form.

Cinnamon Baked Pears

Ingredients:

- Pears
- Ground cinnamon
- A drizzle of honey or sugar substitute

Instructions:

1. Halve pears and remove the core.
2. Sprinkle cinnamon and honey over them.
3. Bake until they're tender and aromatic.

Blueberry Crisp

Ingredients:

- Blueberries
- Rolled oats
- Chopped nuts
- A touch of brown sugar (or sugar substitute)

Instructions:

1. Mix blueberries, oats, nuts, and a small amount of brown sugar.
2. Bake until it's a crunchy, fruity delight.

Chapter 7: Smoothies

In this chapter, we dive into a world of vibrant and delicious smoothie recipes that are not only kidney-friendly but also perfect for those managing diabetes. These smoothies are packed with flavor and wholesome ingredients that will keep your taste buds satisfied and your health in check.

Green Power Smoothie

Ingredients:

- 1 cup fresh spinach leaves
- 1/2 cucumber, peeled and sliced
- 1/2 green apple, cored and chopped
- 1/2 lemon, juiced
- 1 cup water
- Ice cubes (optional)

Instructions:

1. Place all ingredients in a blender.
2. Blend until smooth.
3. Add ice cubes if desired.

4. Serve and enjoy your green power boost!

Berry Blast Smoothie

Ingredients:

- 1 cup mixed berries (strawberries, blueberries, raspberries)
- 1/2 banana
- 1 cup unsweetened almond milk
- 1 tablespoon chia seeds
- Ice cubes (optional)

Instructions:

1. Combine berries, banana, almond milk, and chia seeds in a blender.
2. Blend until smooth.
3. Add ice cubes if you prefer a colder texture.
4. Pour into a glass and savor the berry explosion!

Tropical Paradise Smoothie

Ingredients:

- 1/2 cup pineapple chunks

- 1/2 cup mango chunks
- 1/2 banana
- 1 cup coconut milk
- 1 teaspoon honey (optional)
- Ice cubes (optional)

Instructions:

1. Place pineapple, mango, banana, coconut milk, and honey (if desired) in a blender.
2. Blend until creamy.
3. Add ice cubes for an extra chill.
4. Transport yourself to a tropical paradise with every sip!

Cucumber and Spinach Smoothie

Ingredients:

- 1 cucumber, peeled and sliced
- 1 cup fresh spinach leaves
- 1/2 green apple, cored and chopped
- 1/2 lemon, juiced
- 1 cup water
- Ice cubes (optional)

Instructions:

1. Place cucumber, spinach, green apple, lemon juice, and water in a blender.

2. Blend until smooth.

3. Add ice cubes for extra refreshment.

4. Enjoy the rejuvenating flavors of this unique blend.

Avocado and Kale Smoothie

Ingredients:

- 1 ripe avocado, peeled and pitted
- 1 cup kale leaves
- 1/2 banana
- 1 cup almond milk
- 1 teaspoon honey (optional)
- Ice cubes (optional)

Instructions:

1. Combine avocado, kale, banana, almond milk, and honey (if desired) in a blender.

2. Blend until creamy.

3. Add ice cubes for a cooler treat.

4. Savor the richness and health benefits of this smoothie.

Mango Tango Smoothie

Ingredients:

- 1 cup mango chunks
- 1/2 cup Greek yogurt
- 1/2 banana
- 1/2 orange, juiced
- Ice cubes (optional)

Instructions:

1. Place mango, Greek yogurt, banana, and orange juice in a blender.
2. Blend until velvety.
3. Add ice cubes if you prefer a frosty texture.
4. Dance to the tropical rhythm of this delightful mango tango!

Blueberry Almond Smoothie

Ingredients:

- 1 cup blueberries
- 1/2 cup plain Greek yogurt
- 1/4 cup almonds
- 1/2 teaspoon vanilla extract
- 1 cup almond milk
- Ice cubes (optional)

Instructions:

1. Combine blueberries, Greek yogurt, almonds, vanilla extract, and almond milk in a blender.
2. Blend until smooth.
3. Add ice cubes for extra chill.
4. Sip on this antioxidant-rich blueberry delight!

Chocolate Peanut Butter Smoothie

Ingredients:

- 2 tablespoons unsweetened cocoa powder
- 2 tablespoons peanut butter
- 1 banana

- 1 cup almond milk
- 1 teaspoon honey (optional)
- Ice cubes (optional)

Instructions:

1. Place cocoa powder, peanut butter, banana, almond milk, and honey (if desired) in a blender.
2. Blend until chocolatey perfection.
3. Add ice cubes for a frosty twist.
4. Enjoy the indulgence without guilt.

Coffee Protein Smoothie

Ingredients:

- 1 cup brewed coffee, chilled
- 1/2 cup plain Greek yogurt
- 1 banana
- 1 scoop of your preferred protein powder
- 1 teaspoon honey (optional)
- Ice cubes (optional)

Instructions:

1. Combine chilled coffee, Greek yogurt, banana, protein powder, and honey (if desired) in a blender.
2. Blend until it's a caffeinated delight.
3. Add ice cubes for an extra energizing kick.
4. Enjoy your coffee in a new and healthy way.

Watermelon Mint Smoothie

Ingredients:

- 2 cups fresh watermelon chunks
- 1/2 lime, juiced
- 6-8 fresh mint leaves
- 1 cup coconut water
- Ice cubes (optional)

Instructions:

1. Place watermelon chunks, lime juice, mint leaves, and coconut water in a blender.
2. Blend until it's a refreshing summer sip.
3. Add ice cubes for a cooler experience.
4. Embrace the coolness of watermelon and mint.

Banana Nut Smoothie

Ingredients:

- 2 ripe bananas
- 1/4 cup unsalted mixed nuts
- 1 cup almond milk
- 1/2 teaspoon cinnamon
- 1 teaspoon honey (optional)
- Ice cubes (optional)

Instructions:

1. Combine bananas, mixed nuts, almond milk, cinnamon, and honey (if desired) in a blender.
2. Blend until it's a nutty delight.
3. Add ice cubes for a creamy texture.
4. Enjoy this protein-packed, nutty indulgence.

Strawberry Kiwi Smoothie

Ingredients:

- 1 cup strawberries
- 2 kiwis, peeled and sliced
- 1/2 cup plain Greek yogurt

- 1 teaspoon honey (optional)
- Ice cubes (optional)

Instructions:

1. Place strawberries, kiwis, Greek yogurt, and honey (if desired) in a blender.
2. Blend until it's a fruity symphony.
3. Add ice cubes for a refreshing touch.
4. Sip on this vibrant strawberry-kiwi creation.

Orange Creamsicle Smoothie

Ingredients:

- 2 oranges, peeled and segmented
- 1/2 cup Greek yogurt
- 1/2 banana
- 1 teaspoon vanilla extract
- Ice cubes (optional)

Instructions:

1. Combine orange segments, Greek yogurt, banana, and vanilla extract in a blender.
2. Blend until it's a creamy citrus dream.

3. Add ice cubes for a frosty twist.

4. Relive the nostalgic flavors of a creamsicle.

Spinach and Pineapple Smoothie

Ingredients:

- 2 cups fresh spinach leaves
- 1 cup pineapple chunks
- 1/2 banana
- 1 cup coconut water
- Ice cubes (optional)

Instructions:

1. Place spinach, pineapple, banana, and coconut water in a blender.

2. Blend until it's a green tropical delight.

3. Add ice cubes for an extra cool factor.

4. Boost your day with this green and fruity blend.

Papaya Passion Smoothie

Ingredients:

- 1 cup papaya chunks

- 1/2 cup mango chunks

- 1/2 cup orange juice

- 1/2 lime, juiced

- Ice cubes (optional)

Instructions:

1. Combine papaya, mango, orange juice, and lime juice in a blender.
2. Blend until it's a passionate tropical escape.
3. Add ice cubes for a refreshing kick.
4. Sip on the exotic flavors of papaya and mango.

CONCLUSION

As we reach the conclusion of this culinary journey focused on kidney-friendly diabetic recipes, it's important to reflect on the broader significance of the choices we make in our daily lives. This chapter serves as a reminder that our health and well-being are closely tied to the food we consume.

The journey to better kidney health and diabetes management is a personal one, but it's not a solitary one. It's a path that millions of individuals across the globe are also navigating. In this concluding chapter, we celebrate the collective effort to promote health and share in the accomplishments of countless individuals who have embarked on this journey with determination.

As we part ways, I want to provide some parting thoughts and resources to continue your quest for a healthier lifestyle. Remember, knowledge is power, and the more we understand about our bodies and the food we eat, the better equipped we are to make informed choices.

While this book is a valuable resource, it's just the beginning. Continue to seek knowledge, consult with healthcare professionals, and engage in a supportive community. There are numerous online forums, local support groups, and healthcare providers who are dedicated to helping you along the way. You're not alone in this journey, and the support and guidance available to you are invaluable.

Thank you for taking this step towards improving your kidney health and managing your diabetes. Remember, small changes can yield significant results. Stay committed, stay informed, and continue to savor the delicious, kidney-friendly recipes you've discovered within these pages. Here's to a healthier and more vibrant you!